Erectile Dysfunction

A Step by Step Guide To Naturally Cure ED FAST

By Sean Ward

Sean Ward Copyright © 2016

Table of Contents

Introduction

First and foremost I want to thank you for purchasing the book, "Erectile Dysfunction: A Step by Step Guide To Naturally Cure ED FAST".

In this book you will learn natural and scientific ways to cure ED and maintain erection strength throughout your life, the chapters in this book will show you what has been proven to help improve erectile dysfunction. All will be revealed.

Any man who takes action on the information contained within this book will start to see major changes in the bedroom. Many men are not actually sure what causes erectile dysfunction. It can be very difficult for a man to want to engage in love making but the body will not respond as it once used to.

It is my goal through the pages of this book to educate you on what the natural solutions are to this problem so that you can quickly get on the road to recovery.

Once you are educated on what concrete actions you can take today you will be halfway to solving your ED problem forever. The most important thing to remember is that you need to take real action with the natural methods you will read about in this book!

This book is not a medical journal or am I offering you medical advice. The content in this book is for educational purposes only and you should consult with a licensed physician before taking any actions to increase your testosterone levels.

Thanks again for purchasing this book, I hope you enjoy it!

Chapter 1 Natural Erection Enhancers

If you have googled "natural erection enhancers", you would be amazed at the vast number of men who are concerned about their penis size and the strength of their erections.

The reason so many men are affected is because of some important factors such as; **the rise in obesity**, **poor nutrition choices**, **lack of exercises**, and also because of the rise in men suffering from **low testosterone.**

When men start to notice some problems with their erection strength they naturally will go to the doctor to seek out some help. What usually happens next is your doctor will immediately prescribe you Viagra or

Cialis.

But here's the problem:

Although these medications work they can be very expensive, cause side effects, and not solve the real cause of the problem. For these reasons, a lot of men are now looking for natural erection enhancers that can increase erection strength without the side effects and expenses of prescription drugs.

So if you are one of these people, you should read this chapter as it will inform you about the top natural erection enhancers:

Do Natural Erection Enhancers Really Work?

Natural erection enhancers are very beneficial when compared to their alternatives like Viagra because as mentioned above they don't have many side effects and are a lot cheaper.

Natural erection enhancers are quite different from ordinary erectile dysfunction prescription drugs because they employ natural methods to increase erection, rather than causing biochemical reactions to increase erection strength.

These substances are quite helpful and mimic the effects of chemical drugs, like increasing blood flow through the arteries.

Now before I continue, I just want to say that lifestyle choices do have a massive impact on erection strength.

So it is always important to make sure you are eating the right foods, losing weight, and boosting testosterone alongside using the supplements and foods mentioned below.

List of Male Erection Enhancers

Enough of the chitchat. Let's get down to business. The following is a list of the top male erection enhancers.

This list contains many foods and herbs beneficial for erection strength. So here we go:

1) Garlic

Garlic is known to be very beneficial as a natural testosterone booster. There was an animal study involving rats which showed that garlic can increase testosterone levels, which also leads to better libido and erection strength.

Another benefit of garlic is that it reduces inflammation and blood pressure. As a matter of fact, garlic activates the eNOS system in the body which produces nitric oxide, an enzyme helpful for widening arteries and improving blood flow to your penis.

Garlic consumption has also been shown to reduce blood pressure better than other pharmaceutical products and high blood pressure is one of the major causes of erectile dysfunction and weak erections.

Another interesting human study also showed that when garlic is combined with a Vitamin C supplement, there is a massive 200% increase in nitric oxide levels along with a decrease in systolic and diastolic blood pressure levels.

2) Korean Ginseng

Ginseng root was one of the first herbs that received mass media coverage since the early 1990s. It was said that this wonder herb improved concentration, enhanced memory, and increased sexual desire.

However, one of the most important uses of ginseng for centuries has been as an adaptogen, which basically means that it can help to reduce stress and keep the adrenal system balanced.

The reason this is important is because stress can increase blood pressure and can also lower testosterone levels which are two of the major causes of weak erections.

It gets better:

Not only does Korean Ginseng reduce stress but it also improves nitric oxide levels in the body.

In fact, there was a study done in Korea involving 45 men who were suffering from erectile dysfunction.

After only 8 weeks of taking Ginseng, the men reported improvements in erection strength and sexual satisfaction.

There was also another study done that involved 60 men suffering from ED who took 100mg of Ginseng 3 times a day.

The researchers found that after 12 weeks the men had marked improvements in being able to maintain a hard erection.

3) Pycnogenol

Pycnogenol is a plant extract that is derived from the bark of the french maritime pine tree in France. The reason that Pycnogenol is a great natural erection enhancer is because it has the power to increase nitric oxide production.

How it does this is by increasing the enzyme NOS (nitric oxide synthase) which leads to more nitric oxide in the body.

A study that involved men taking 180 mg of Pycnogenol resulted in improved vasodilation and increased arterial expansion. This increased blood flow will improve erection strength and help men who suffer from erectile dysfunction.

There was also a study that investigated the effect of taking 40mg's of Pycnogenol along with 1700mgs of Arginine 3 times daily.

After just 3 months of this regime, the men reported that they were now experiencing erections again.

4) Pomegranate

Pomegranates are quite beneficial for erectile strength and they can do wonders for your health too. Calling them a Natural Viagra might not be that untrue.

If you don't believe it, just look at the different studies which have proven its benefits for hormonal health and circulation.

An Israeli study showed that long-term consumption of pomegranate is associated with an increase in nitric oxide levels and a drop in blood pressure levels. There is also a decrease in arterial plaque and reduction in bad "LDL-cholesterol."

Moreover, another human study showed that daily pomegranate consumption increases testosterone levels by 24%.

Bottom Line:

Pomegranate can help men who are having problems with erection strength and can also help men suffering with erectile dysfunction.

5) L-arginine

L-arginine is an amino acid found in meat and dairy products. It can also be created in the laboratory.

Citrulline, however, is an amino acid that can be found in watermelon that transforms to Arginine in the kidneys.

There are many studies to show how arginine can increase nitric oxide. Arginine is basically a vasodilator, which means it expands blood vessels and improves blood flow. All the studies show that L-Arginine increases nitric oxide and blood flow.

The bottom line is that Arginine or Citrulline is known as a safe treatment for erectile dysfunction in humans.

6) Nitrate-Rich Leafy Greens

What you need to know about dietary nitrates is that they are converted into nitrites by tongue-bacteria present in the gut and the bacteria there converts the nitrites into precious nitric oxide.

This relaxes the arteries and helps increase blood circulation, which also improves the circulation and blood flow to the penis resulting in better erections.

There are some foods rich in nitrates:

Spinach, Kale, Iceberg Lettuce, Beets, Arugula, Celery, Collard Greens, Cabbage, Radishes and Swiss chard.

7) Zinc

Everyone has heard of zinc and most people know about its beneficial effects on the body, but the question is whether it enhances erections?

Here's what you need to know:

There have been numerous scientific studies to prove that Zinc increases testosterone and significantly improves libido in men.

So for that reason, it won't hurt to add zinc in your diet by eating foods like pumpkin seeds, oysters, nuts, shellfish, egg yolk, and beans.

Boosting testosterone by increasing zinc levels is going to have a positive effect on erection strength.

Now you know a list of some natural erection enhancers. The main goal of all these natural erection enhancers is to increase erection strength.

As mentioned earlier in this article there are definitely some foods for harder erections that if eaten regularly can help any man improve his erection strength.

If you follow the advice in this article you will never have to worry about erection strength.

So let's now get to the next chapter.

Chapter 2 Maca Root Benefits For Men

In this chapter let us talk about the recently popular plants grown in the North America. You might have not heard about it, but it has now become a popular herb and food. We're talking about maca root.

The main reason for the wide usage of maca root is because it enhances male libido and sexual performance. There are tons of benefits for using this root but here we'll discuss the benefit for males only. So let us jump right into it.

What is Maca root?

The scientific names of maca root are Lepidium Peruvianum or Lepidium meyenii. It has been used for quite some time for its energy enhancing and mood stabilizing properties. It's composed of many powerful ingredients like amino acids, vitamins, phytonutrients, fatty acids and vitamins. Maca root is prized because of its benefits like boosting hormones, helping with digestion, fertility and increasing energy levels.

Benefits of Maca Root for Men

Maca root has a long list of health benefits for men, most of which are aphrodisiac (increasing sexual performance). But you should always consult your healthcare professional before self-treating with maca root.

Some major health benefits of maca root for men include:

1. Male sexual health:

The Memorial Sloan Kettering Cancer Center has noted that many human and animal studies have indicated that maca roots may actually help in increasing male libido and sexual performance. A study published in the 2009 edition of "Andrologia", found that men who took maca supplements for three straight months had an increase in sexual functioning in the 8th and 12th week. No increase was seen in the placebo group.

There were two groups who received the supplement; one received 1500 mg daily and the other received 3000 mg daily. It was noted that the amount taken didn't influence the desire level.

After a year, scientists wanted to know whether the elevated mood was the reason that maca had positive effect in enhancing male sexual functioning. To check this, males between the ages of 15 and 30 were given 1500 mg maca, 3000 mg maca and placebo.

The tests were done after four, eight and twelve months to see how the individuals felt about their sexual desire and anxiety. The men noted an improvement in sexual desire after eight weeks.

2. Maca Root and Male Fertility:

Maca root can improve fertility in men. It improves fertility by increasing the sperm production in men. A study was done by J. Nieto and his colleagues which was published in the 2006 issue of "Andrologia in which it was found that maca root increases the sperm count just one day after treatment. In the study, the subjects were given 2 grams of maca for 12 days and the sperm counts were tested after every two days.

The results showed that there was an increase in the sperm count one day after treatment and the sperm production also increased after the seventh day.

Maca root can help in treating male infertility but more studies are still needed to verify it. A study was performed by J.Rubio and his colleagues which was published in the July 2006 edition of "Food and Chemical Toxicology" which showed that maca has the ability to reverse the male infertility caused by chemical exposure. The subjects were tested for this study were given 0.8, 0.16 and 0.24 mg of lead acetate for 35 days.

The subjects were divided into two groups; the first was the control group and the other received maca for last 18 days. The results showed that the subjects which were given maca had reversed their lead-induced infertility and increased their sperm production.

3. Sexual dysfunction and Prostate Health:

A recent study supporting the maca is beneficial for sexual dysfunction was performed in Italy where the researchers conducted a double-blind study. About fifty men who had mild erection were selected for the study. Half of them were given 2400 mg maca root and the other half were in placebo. The results were viewed after 12 weeks.

These results showed that men who took maca supplements had an increase in the International Index of Erectile Function (IIEF-5) as compared to men in the placebo group. The scientists concluded that maca supplements are quite beneficial for men with mild erectile dysfunction.

Maca root also benefits prostate health. The color of maca matters when it comes to prostate health. It is available in yellow, black and red forms and researchers compared the impact of each on prostate size of rats with induced prostatic hyperplasia (a health condition in which prostate is enlarged).

The results showed that the red form has prostate-reducing effects whereas yellow has a mild effect and black has no effect at all.

4. Increasing Energy:

Maca root has the ability to increase energy levels in men. It also increases stamina. There is evidence that athletes have used maca supplements in place of anabolic steroids for enhanced performance. You should include maca extracts in your diet if you feel tired most of the time. A small amount can do wonders for your health.

5. Regulating Hormones:

Maca contains a variety of amino acids, which function as the building blocks of hormones. Research has shown that the hormones of men who take maca on regular basis are balanced. Maca doesn't create hormones but function as the building blocks for hormones.

6. General Health:

Maca root improves the overall health of men in many ways. It provides iron to the body and restores the red blood cells which help against cardiovascular diseases and anemia. It also keeps the teeth and bones healthy and helps in the quick healing of wounds. You would notice an increase in muscle mass if you use maca extracts in combination with a good workout.

But you should be careful while using maca if you have cancer related to testicles. People with liver issues and high blood pressure should also consult a doctor before using maca.

How to take Maca?

Maca extracts can be consumed in a variety of forms like it can be added in recipes and used in tablet form. You should consume about 1,500 to 3,000 mg of maca in capsule form daily.

You can also intake maca in loose powder form. You should start taking 1 teaspoon per day and increase up to 3 to 6 teaspoons daily. You should keep this schedule for three to six months.

Conclusion

As you can see there are many Maca root benefits for men especially when it comes to enhancing libido.

If your libido needs a boost give Maca a try and I'm sure you will be happy with the results.

Chapter 3 Citrulline Benefits For Men

This chapter is going to look at some of the benefits of citrulline for men and look at how supplementing with citrulline can improve erection strength and boost nitric oxide.

Citrulline is one of the few supplements which has a lot of medical and therapeutic benefits that make it a great supplement for men to take.

This supplement is thought to be beneficial for men for a number of reasons, the most important of which is that it increases nitric oxide levels in the body.

For those of you who don't know what citrulline is, it is an amino acid and supplement used for sports performance and cardiovascular health. But there is much more to this supplement that you might not know. So read this chapter to know more about citrulline:

Citrulline – A brief Introduction

The word citrulline actually comes from the latin word citrullus, meaning watermelon. You can increase the amount of citrulline in the body by eating foods like watermelon, garlic, cucumbers, onions, and milk protein.

Citrulline is converted into arginine in the body which is the amino acid responsible for producing nitric oxide. What research is now showing is that citrulline can increase nitric oxide levels better than taking arginine directly.

The reason for this is because 50% of arginine is converted to ornithine in the liver. This means that when arginine is ingested only half of it will be converted into nitric oxide. However citrulline is not metabolized by the liver but instead goes to the kidneys where it is easily converted into arginine.

Citrulline helps to reduce fatigue and improve endurance levels for both aerobic and non-aerobic exercises. It also used for erectile dysfunction, diabetes, bodybuilding, and high blood pressure.

Citrulline Benefits for Men

There are a number of benefits of citrulline for men, which have been mentioned below:

Citrulline Promotes Erectile Strength

Probably one of the biggest benefits of citrulline is the hardness factor and how it can increase erectile strength.

Citrulline is somewhat new in the erectile supplement market because researchers were previously concentrated on a similar supplement, named L-Arginine that proved to be beneficial for improving testosterone levels.

L-Arginine was also being studied for it benefits on nitric oxide production. However, what the researchers found was that Arginine had to be taken in very high doses to have any effect and for some men this could be dangerous.

There has been less research done on citrulline but recent studies are now starting to discover all the benefits of citrulline.

There was even a study that showed how citrulline outperformed arginine at increasing nitric oxide production in the body.

Here are some more studies which show the benefits of Citrulline:

A study was recently done in which 24 men with erectile dysfunction received a placebo for one month, followed by a 1.5 g/day dose of citrulline daily for another month. The ages of men were between 50 and 70 years and they reported no side effects.

The researchers concentrated on those individuals who had a reduction of penile rigidity but still were able to achieve vaginal penetration. None of the patients involved in the study had any cardiovascular, psychiatric or nervous disorders.

The results were better than expected. During the placebo treatment, only 2 out of the 24 patients reported an increase in erectile strength but when the patients switched to citrulline, 12 out of 24 patients had an increase in penile strength.

So, this study proved that citrulline increased penile hardness by 50%.

Another study was done on rats with erectile dysfunction. The main aim of the study was to find out if citrulline supplementation improves erection strength in rats with erectile dysfunction.

The rats were divided into three groups; the sham-operated rats which were the control group, the arteriogenic erectile dysfunction rats and the erectile dysfunction rats who received 2% citrulline supplementation.

The citrulline water was given to the rats for three weeks from 1 week after the surgery period. The erectile function was evaluated about 4 weeks after surgery. Then the penises were resected and the nitrogen oxide levels were measured.

The results showed that the levels of nitric oxide were the lowest in the control group whereas they were highest in the ED group receiving citrulline.

This proves that oral supplementation of citrulline is a good therapy to improve erectile dysfunction.

There has always been a debate about whether citrulline is better or L-arginine. A study was recently done to find out whether citrulline can be used as an alternative to L-arginine.

It was a double-blind, randomized and placebo-controlled study in which the subjects received six different doses of placebo, citrulline, and arginine. The pharmacokinetic parameters were evaluated after 1 week of supplementation.

The results were obtained and observed which clearly showed that citrulline increases NO levels in the same ratio as L-arginine. So, citrulline can be used as an alternative to L-arginine for erectile strength.

These studies clearly show that citrulline is helpful at increasing nitric oxide in the body which can help men with erection problems.

Intestinal Absorption

Citrulline is absorbed in the intestine at a much higher level as compared to its counterparts, like L-arginine and this results in higher plasma levels.

Numerous sodium-dependent transporters are responsible for its absorption. So, in contrast to L-arginine, citrulline is better absorbed in the intestine and may be a better absorptive material than L-arginine.

Cardiovascular Health

There are several studies which show that the intake of citrulline may improve heart and arterial health.

In fact, a study was recently published in the cardiology Journal which involved people with heart failure.

The study found out that citrulline supplementation for two months improves performance on the treadmill and lowers blood pressure; this leads to better heart function. The arterial walls of the arteries also become less stiff, which improves heart health.

Improves Learning and Memory

Citrulline has quite a few interactions with memory because it increases nitric oxide and improves blood flow through the arteries.

Citrulline has found to be at a higher concentration in the hippocampus of trained rats as compared to untrained rats.

This alone proves that citrulline is helpful in enhancing memory. But more research is still needed to give a conclusive statement.

Citrulline Dosage

Citrulline is abundantly found in watermelon with 290 mg in an average cup of watermelon. There are different scientific reviews written about the exact dosage of citrulline.

There has been some research done in Germany that showed that a 3 grams dose of Citrulline produced the largest increase in both Arginine and Nitric Oxide levels.

To get enough citrulline you can consume a few cups of watermelon each day or you could take it in powder form.

Conclusion

Now you know the health benefits of citrulline for men.

From promoting erectile strength to cardiovascular health to improving memory, citrulline is a great supplement for any man to take.

Chapter 4 Best Vitamins and Exercises for Erectile Dysfunction

Do you know what the best vitamins for erectile dysfunction are? Do you know which supplements can increase erection strength?

In this chapter, we are going to cover what vitamins have been scientifically proven to increase erection strength in men.

The vitamins mentioned below will not only improve erection strength but will also increase testosterone and nitric oxide production.

We will also be discussing some exercises that will improve blood flow to the groin area helping to improve erections.

Research from the Natural Institutes of Health tells us that 15 to 25 percent of 65-year-old men are affected by erectile dysfunction and 5 percent of men who are 40 are also affected.

But if you provide your body with the right vitamins to increase nitric oxide and blood flow you will not have to suffer from erectile dysfunction any longer.

Let's now dive into some of the best vitamins for erectile dysfunction.

Supplements That Increase Erection Strength

Vitamin C For Erectile Dysfunction

Vitamin C has to be first on the list of the best vitamins for erectile dysfunction. There is a lot of research to show how Vitamin C can increase nitric oxide production in the body and studies to show how it protects nitric oxide from being attacked by free radicals.

In fact, research from a 2010 study by Reproductive Partners Medical Group showed that Vitamin C and Calcium helped the pathways that lead to improvements in nitric oxide production which are very important for men wanting to cure erectile dysfunction.

The reason that nitric oxide is so important to erection strength is because nitric oxide improves blood flow and oxygen delivery to every area of your body including the penis. To help improve nitric oxide it is a good idea to stop smoking and be moderate in alcohol consumption.

There is now research that shows that when 2 grams of vitamin C is taken with 4 garlic tablets (containing 13.2 mg of alliin and 6 mg of allicin) the levels of nitric oxide increased by an amazing 200% and blood pressure dropped to levels not even achieved by regular medication.

This shows that saving money and supplementing with Vitamin C and Garlic can be a great way to improve erectile dysfunction.

Vitamin D For Erectile Dysfunction

Vitamin D is actually not a vitamin but is, in fact, a hormone. This hormone has been shown to improve testosterone levels and improve nitric oxide production in the body.

Without Vitamin D there will be no nitric oxide released in the body and without nitric oxide, you can say goodbye to strong erections.

But Vitamin D has other benefits for general health aside from hormonal health and nitric oxide production.

According to the acclaimed Vitamin D expert, Dr. Michael Holick this vitamin has the greatest power of all the vitamins he has researched to improve human health.

With all the studies that have been done on Vitamin D what researchers have found is that men with Vitamin D deficiencies have lower nitric oxide levels and lower testosterone levels.

The combination of low nitric oxide levels and low testosterone is going to have a negative impact on erection strength

Lets now look at the studies that show why low levels of Vitamin D can lead to erection problems and low testosterone.

- A study done by the University of Milan showed that men with erectile dysfunction had 20% lower levels of Vitamin D compared with men who had no problems with erection strength.

- This study that involved 1362 men showed that when the subjects took a supplement of Vitamin D there was a significant increase in testosterone levels.
- This study showed that men with adequate levels of Vitamin D had high levels of testosterone compared with men who were deficient in Vitamin D.
- A great way to get Vitamin D is to take a High Vitamin Butter Oil/Fermented Cod Liver Oil supplement.

Vitamin E For Erectile Dysfunction

Vitamin E is another great vitamin for erectile dysfunction. The reason Vitamin E is important is because it's a powerful antioxidant which can help to increase the levels of nitric oxide in the body.

The increase in nitric oxide will help blood flow throughout the body which will increase erection strength.

Vitamin E is also great for promoting arousal in men. The way Vitamin E promote arousal is by boosting the production of prostaglandins which are compounds with hormone-like effects. Vitamin E has also been shown to protect cells from damage and protects the heart from damage.

It is well-known fact that anything that keeps the heart healthy will also lead to a healthy sex life.

Here are some studies to show how Vitamin E is one of the best supplements to increase erection strength.

- A study concluded that antioxidant therapy with Vitamin E improved age-associated erectile dysfunction.
- Another study showed that 4 weeks of taking 1000 i.u. of Vitamin E increased nitric oxide production and blood flow in the body.
- Lastly, another study showed that supplementation with Vitamin E significantly increased testosterone in human subjects and male rats.

To make sure you are getting enough Vitamin E consume foods such as nuts, seeds, green leafy vegetables and fish.

If you want to get a good quality Vitamin E supplement look for one with natural tocopherols.

Citrulline For Erectile Dysfunction

Citrulline is a very powerful supplement to take for anyone wanting to find a natural cure for erectile dysfunction. Citrulline is converted into L-Arginine which is an amino acid that makes nitric oxide in the body.

You might be thinking that if L-Arginine makes nitric oxide which helps erections then why not take L-Arginine instead of Citrulline. However what studies are now showing is that Citrulline is even more powerful at improving erections than L-Arginine so let's see why this is the case.

The reason that L-Arginine is not as effective as Citrulline is because when it is ingested nearly 50% is converted into ornithine by the enzyme arginase in the liver. This means that half of L-Arginine will not be converted into nitric oxide but instead, will be metabolized in the liver.

This is where Citrulline is so useful because unlike L-Arginine it's not metabolized in the liver but instead goes into the kidneys where it is easily transformed into L-Arginine. All the studies conclude that Citrulline raises both nitric oxide and levels of L-Arginine in the blood more dramatically than taking L-Arginine alone.

Let's take a look at the scientific proof that Citrulline helps erectile dysfunction.

- A study showed that Citrulline supplementation increased erection hardness in men suffering from erectile dysfunction.
- Another study showed that Arginine levels in the body increased by 22% through the intake of Citrulline.
- Lastly, a study showed that Citrulline supplementation increased nitric oxide in 20 healthy volunteers.

The best dietary source of Citrulline is watermelon. One cup of watermelon contains around 250 milligrams of Citrulline making it a great and easy way to improve erections.

Now let us look at other ways to increase erection strength

Best Exercises For Erectile Dysfunction

When it comes to improving erection strength one thing we have to concentrate on is improving blood flow. So with that in mind here are some of the best exercises for erectile dysfunction that will improve blood flow to the penis.

Core Exercises

Doing core exercises are a great way to improve erection strength because when the core region is exercised blood supply is increased not only in the core area but also to the groin.

Leg raises are a great way to achieve this.

Bodyweight Squats

Bodyweight squats are another great exercise that will improve erection strength because they improve circulation in the body and help blood supply to the groin area.

They also work one of the biggest muscle groups in the body resulting in a natural boost of testosterone.

Kegel Exercises for Men

Kegel exercises are a very powerful way to boost blood flow to the penis. They can also help men to last longer when having sex.

Action Plan To Cure Erectile Dysfunction

Here is a clear plan of action to naturally cure ED

- Make sure you are getting adequate levels of the best vitamins for erectile dysfunction discussed above.

- Eat foods that improve erectile performance.

- Include some of the exercises mentioned in this article that will help blood supply to the groin area.

- Naturally increase your testosterone levels.

- Include some powerful natural pde5 inhibitors into your diet.

Conclusion

I hope this article has helped you understand some of the best vitamins for erectile dysfunction and how getting adequate levels of these vitamins can help to improve erectile health.

Chapter 5 Apple Cider Vinegar for Erectile Dysfunction

Did you know that about 90% of people over the age of 50 suffer from erectile dysfunction?

This may sound really depressing but it definitely doesn't have to be this way and in this chapter, I am going to be exploring the strong link between apple cider vinegar and erectile dysfunction.

I will also be taking a look at all the numerous health benefits of consuming apple cider vinegar.

There are many natural treatments for erectile dysfunction and as you are about to find out one of the best natural treatments is the use of apple cider vinegar.

So if you want to know more about the link between apple cider vinegar and erectile dysfunction keep reading.

Erectile Dysfunction and Causes

Before I go any further, you should know that erectile dysfunction isn't a disease in itself but is a symptom of many other problems within the body.

The most common medical conditions which cause erectile dysfunction are high blood pressure, high cholesterol, depression and prostate disease.

Two other factors that contribute to erectile dysfunction are low testosterone levels and poor blood circulation.

All the health problems listed above lead to lower testosterone levels and poor blood circulation. So, if you have any of these problems, you are going to be more prone to erectile dysfunction and impotence.

Apple Cider Vinegar and Erectile Dysfunction

Apple cider vinegar can be very helpful in dealing with erectile dysfunction and the way it helps is by improving the health problems mentioned above like high cholesterol levels, high blood pressure, diabetes etc.

These conditions affect your health and blood flow to the penis, which is necessary to get a firm hard erection.

Apple cider vinegar has antibacterial, antifungal and antiviral properties. Other than this, many important minerals and vitamins are present in apple cider vinegar that can help to fight erectile dysfunction.

The important minerals and vitamins present in apple cider vinegar include Vitamin A, Vitamin B, Vitamin B2, Vitamin B6, Vitamin C, Vitamin P, calcium, chlorine, copper, iron, magnesium, sodium, Sulphur etc.

How Apple Cider Vinegar Helps Erectile Dysfunction

The great thing about curing erectile dysfunction using apple cider vinegar is that it works quickly in the body. You can notice a rise in your sexual desire after just one day, but mostly it occurs after two to three days.

Apple cider vinegar reduces and repairs the nerve fibers and blood vessels around the penis. It can also reduce the swelling of the prostate gland which can lead to better erections.

Recent researchers have also suggested that it can increase testosterone levels and facilitate weight loss, which eventually can help in curing erectile dysfunction.

4 Ways Apple Cider Vinegar Cures Erectile Dysfunction

Here are 4 ways that apple cider vinegar can help erectile dysfunction

1) Apple Cider Vinegar Lowers Blood Sugar

High blood sugar levels are linked to diabetes which can weaken the blood vessels in the body include the area around the penis. There are a **bunch of studies** in which the effect of apple cider vinegar on blood sugar levels and blood pressure were measured.

Diabetes was induced in rats by injecting them with an injection of streptozotocin. Both the normal and diabetic rats were fed with apple cider vinegar for 4 consecutive weeks. The results were obtained which showed that the administration of apple cider vinegar in diabetic rats lowered blood sugar levels.

Moreover, it improved lipid profile too and lowered blood pressure too. All these factors are linked to erectile dysfunction.

A study was done recently to find out whether the intake of apple cider vinegar during bedtime reduces the glucose concentrations after waking. The subjects of the study included 7 people, four men and 7 women who were diagnosed with type 2 diabetes. The participants of the study followed a 24-hour diet with 2 tbsp apple cider vinegar before bedtime daily.

The results of the study showed that apple cider vinegar reduces about 6% of the fasting glucose. These results clearly indicate that apple cider vinegar is beneficial in treating type 2 diabetes.

2) Apple Cider Vinegar Lowers Cholesterol

Apple cider vinegar contains an antioxidant known as Chlorogenic acid, which keeps the cholesterol particles away from the heart and thus can prevent heart disease. And any kind of vascular disease is going to be bad for erectile health.

A study was done recently to find out the effect of Chlorogenic acid on low-density lipoproteins. For the study, the effect of Chlorogenic acid on LDL cholesterol was researched.

The results of the study showed that Chlorogenic acid reduced the LDL levels, which reduces the lipid peroxidation; this helps to prevent heart diseases and erectile dysfunction.

3) Apple Cider Vinegar Speeds Up Weight Loss

Apple cider vinegar has been used for many centuries as a weight loss aid. Even a small amount of apple cider vinegar can function as a very powerful appetite suppressant.

The glucose regulating properties of apple cider vinegar can also help to keep your weight in check.

Your body fat contains an enzyme called aromatase which converts your testosterone into estrogen so any reduction in body weight will lead to more free testosterone.

Apple cider vinegar also speeds up the metabolic process, which leads to weight loss.

4) Apple Cider Vinegar Improves Insulin Sensitivity

A study was done recently by the American Diabetes Association of Arizona University to find out the effect of apple cider vinegar on insulin sensitivity in patients suffering from Type 2 diabetes.

The number of subjects for the study was 20, which included patients who were either insulin sensitive or suffering from type 2 diabetes. The subjects were given either a placebo drink or vinegar drink (containing apple cider vinegar).

The vinegar intake in the subjects led to improvements in insulin sensitivity. This data indicates that vinegar can improve insulin sensitivity.

By reducing the insulin levels, apple cider vinegar also prevents artery damage. And artery damage is a big cause of erectile dysfunction.

Other Health Benefits of Apple Cider Vinegar

Curing erectile dysfunction is just one of the many benefits of apple cider vinegar. Some other health benefits are mentioned below:

- Apple Cider Vinegar is high in acetic acid which is very beneficial for the body.

- Apple Cider Vinegar regulates the pH levels of the skin.

- Apple Cider Vinegar acts as a good detoxifying agent.

- Apple Cider Vinegar can help the body in getting rid of candida.

- Apple Cider Vinegar has antimicrobial properties and has the ability to kill different types of bacteria.

- Apple Cider Vinegar has protective effects against cancer.

Apple Cider Vinegar Dosage for Erectile Dysfunction

The great thing about apple cider vinegar is that you can consume it in a few different ways.

You can simply put a tablespoon of apple cider vinegar into a pint of water and add a small teaspoon of honey for taste.

You could also make a detox drink which includes apple cider vinegar, lemon juice, cinnamon, cayenne pepper and stevia.

Another good way to consume apple cider vinegar is to add a tablespoon of it to salads alongside some testosterone boosting olive oil.

When first starting out it's a good idea to take one tablespoon of apple cider vinegar each day and slowly work your way up from there.

The best quality organic cider vinegar to consume is without a doubt from the legendary late Paul Bragg.

Conclusion

As you can see from the evidence there is a big link between apple cider vinegar and erectile dysfunction.

You can easily incorporate into your diet by using it as a salad dressing or as mentioned by drinking it with water. And if you combine apple cider vinegar with some foods proven to **increase erection strength** you will be pleasantly surprised with the results.

With all of the many health benefits, that apple cider can give it really makes sense to incorporate it into your life.

Chapter 6 Foods that Boost Nitric Oxide in the Body

Why have a chapter on foods that contain nitric oxide?

Well, the reason we want to make sure we are consuming Nitric Oxide rich food is because the Nitric Oxide molecule is known to be a potent and natural vasodilator.

What this means for you is it will improve the ability to circulate blood around the body by helping to dilate blood vessels and expand arteries.

In a nutshell, Nitric Oxide will improve blood flow and circulation in the body that will contribute to every area of our health including heart health, brain health, and sexual health.

This is due to the increased oxygen, nutrients and red blood cells that come with increased circulation.

The knock on effect of this is that blood vessels in your penis will start to open up and relax allowing blood to flow inside leading to a nice firm erection.

Interestingly one of the ways Viagra works is by slowing the breakdown of Nitric Oxide which then allows levels to start to increase in the body. So anything we can do to increase Nitric Oxide will lead to stronger erections.

A side benefit of this is when we do have an erection our testosterone will be boosted leading to an increased libido for yes you guessed it more erections.

Ok so now we are going to cover the foods that contain nitric oxide. All of these foods have been shown to be rich in nitrates which your body will then go about converting to Nitric Oxide.

So let's dive right in

Foods High in Nitric Oxide

1. Dark Chocolate

Several studies have shown how dark chocolate can increase nitric oxide and blood flow in the body. The research shows that polyphenols found in dark chocolate can reduce oxidative stress and help the body produce more nitric oxide.

2. *Watermelon*

Sometimes called natures viagra watermelon contains an abundant amount of L-Citrulline which is then converted into Nitric Oxide in the body. This ability of watermelon to raise nitric oxide has been proven in numerous studies.

3. Pomegranate

Pomegranate has gained a massive amount of research showing its ability to improve cardiovascular health. This ability to improve cardiovascular health and blood pressure is in large part due to how its compounds help to boost nitric oxide and blood flow through the body.

4. Arugula

The reason arugula is so powerful as a nitric oxide booster is because it contains more nitrates that any other vegetable out there.

5. Beet Juice

The reason that we want to be consuming beet juice is because firstly beets are known to increase nitric oxide but secondly they also help to lower estrogen by acting as a methylator.

And by helping to keep estrogen levels low our testosterone levels will start to increase.

6. Spinach

Spinach contains an abundant amount of nitrates and a study was done at Karolinska Institute in Stockholm that showed that adding nitrates to men's diets lead to muscles becoming more stronger and efficient so Popeye really did know his stuff.

7. Oranges

Oranges help with the production of nitric oxide by the high amounts of Vitamin C they contain protecting nitric oxide from being attacked by free radicals thereby keeping nitric oxide levels high.

8. Walnuts

Walnuts pack a potent dose of the amino acid L-Arginine and one of the key functions of this amino acid is to convert into nitric oxide.

9. Salmon

Salmon is a very good food to eat for overall health with its high concentration of essential fatty acids but the mighty salmon also contains a dose of Co-enzyme

Q10 and this enzyme has been shown in studies to protect your nitric oxide and increase it in the body.

10. Kale

If you are a vegetarian or vegan but still want the benefits that Co-enzyme Q10 has on nitric oxide production then Kale is something you want to have handy in the kitchen as it contains a good amount of Co-enzyme Q10 and it also is one of the most nutrient dense foods you can eat.

Conclusion

If you are serious enough about increasing your nitric oxide levels try to add some of these nutrient packed foods into your diet. This will lead to levels of nitric oxide rising and you will reap all the benefits to heart health and also erectile health.

Please remember that as your levels start to increase by adding these foods high in nitric oxide to your diet you will be improving how your body performs in just about every way you can think of.

Because along with testosterone nitric oxide is very important for men's health so don't waste no time and get these foods down you ASAP.

Chapter 7 How To Increase Sex Drive in Men Over 40

This chapter is going to look into how to increase sex drive in men over 40 and how this can be done with some lifestyle changes.

Did you know that your sex drive decreases with age? The main reason behind this is that the production of HGH (Human Growth Hormone) and testosterone hormones decrease as you age.

A man's sex drive peaks at 30 years and starts declining after that. So you need to take strong measures to boost your testosterone levels and sex drive after that.

Sex Drive in Men Over 40

Research has shown that most of the people who go to the doctor with their libido issues are over the age 40. They have different complaints like they feel less interested in sex compared to how they used to or they just don't feel a lot of sexual energy.
You should know here that getting your sex drive back isn't all about sex. You need to know that sexual desire is related to the energy and vitality flowing in your body.

There are many natural ways that men can boost their sex drive and these are discussed below.

1) Diet

Diet plays a major role in sex drive. Your sex drive is bound to be lower if you don't eat properly. The best way to counter the effect of diet is to eat the foods that boost your sexual health. The following are some quality foods for boosting your sexual drive:

Grapes

You should eat a bunch of grapes on a daily basis to boost your sex drive. They contain resveratrol that increases sperm production and testosterone levels. Researchers recently found that grapes can boost your testosterone levels and improve your sperm motility.

Tuna

Some people avoid tuna because of its smell but you should know that it is rich in Vitamin D which is great for boosting testosterone. A study found that the vitamin D found in tuna can increase testosterone levels by 90%. A can of tuna contains about 100% of the daily Vitamin D intake.

Oysters

Oysters are great for increasing a person's sex drive because they are rich in zinc. Zinc is a very important mineral for improving muscle performance and boosting growth hormone levels. Research has proven that zinc helps in boosting testosterone levels in the body.

Garlic

Garlic is beneficial in boosting a person's sex drive. The main reason is that it triggers the release of luteinzing hormone, which has been shown to boost testosterone levels in the body.

Both garlic and onions contain a chemical known as diallyl disulfide which increases sperm concentration in the testes.

Eggs

As I have said many times eggs are one of the best foods you can eat to boost your testosterone levels. A famous nutritionist Kim Pearson says that the yolk in eggs is very beneficial for boosting testosterone levels. You shouldn't worry about your heart because eating three eggs a day doesn't affect cholesterol levels.

2) Water

Water is also very helpful for improving libido because the blood contains about 90% water. You should drink about six to eight glasses of water to keep your energy levels high.

Another reason that water is important for libido is because studies have shown that even mild dehydration can significantly increase the stress hormone cortisol.

And because cortisol lowers testosterone it really is important to stay hydrated throughout the day to keep cortisol down. The best way to increase water intake is to drink water between meals and make sure to drink it from a glass bottle because we want to avoid plastic bottles that contain xenoestrogens.

3) Cut Stress

People over 40 stress more and as mentioned above the stress hormone has the ability to lower the male sex drive because it can lower testosterone. Stress keeps you alert and focused on potential threats but when your body is in this state the arteries can narrow.

When the arteries narrow this can lead to restricted blood flow in the body that can contribute to erectile dysfunction. Short term stress can become long term because of daily worries. So this can seriously switch off the sex drive.

You should adopt the following ways to lower stress in your life.

- Exercise is quite beneficial in lowering stress levels as long as you do not overtrain and increase the stress hormone cortisol. You can also do exercises which help you relax and recover like yoga.

- Try not to skip too many meals. When you skip eating regular meals over a long period of time the body stresses and goes in 'famine' mood. This means that less energy is reserved for sex.

- Never overwork yourself. Some people work too much and sleep too little which increase stress. So you should know your limits and have proper work-free periods.

- Meditation can help you learn the skill of being able to relax at will. It can also help you to achieve quality deep sleep that will increase testosterone levels.

4) Exercise and Lose Body Fat
Exercise is really important for anyone wanting to boost sex drive. Burning body fat through regular exercise will help boost your testosterone levels like

nothing else. The reason for this is because inside of body fat, the enzyme aromatase is abundant and this enzyme converts your testosterone into estrogen very efficiently.

The way to lower body fat is to do 3 full body workouts each week and on your days off do some light aerobic activity like walking, low-intensity jogging or a bike ride to keep your activity levels up and burn calories.

5) Set The Mood

When you start to feel your sex drive becoming stronger now is the time to concentrate on setting the mood for sex. In a partially stable relationship, sex is sometimes considered as the last activity of the day. But you should give a lot of attention to having sex.

Take some time to set the scene and spend some time together before having sex like having a meal. You should make your wife/girlfriend the sole focus for one evening in a week.

You should also create a relaxing environment and make sure that you aren't disturbed during this time. You should also change the way you have sex with your partner each time so it doesn't become boring and is always exciting.

6) Sleep

Research has found a very real link between sleep and sex drive. The main reason behind this is that the body makes testosterone and growth hormone during deep sleep. So do what you can to get some deep sleep of between 7 to 9 hours every night. The time from 10pm to 1am are the three most important hours for sleep. So it is advisable to go to bed by 11 pm.

If you have trouble getting deep sleep you could try relaxation techniques a few hours before bed or you could try the calming herb ashwagandha to get quality sleep. Don't do anything which disrupts your sleep. You should also have calmness and quietness in your bedroom. A good idea to stop outside noise and interference is to put earplugs in your ears when you go to bed.

Conclusion

I hope this chapter about how to increase sex drive in men over 40 has given you some useful advice on the lifestyle changes you can make right away that will have a positive impact on your wellbeing and sexual energy.

www.ingramcontent.com/pod-product-compliance
Lightning Source LLC
Chambersburg PA
CBHW071247280526
45788CB00004B/1613